CONTENTS

POSITIVE AFFIRMATIONS FOR HEALTH ANXIETY

50 Empowering Affirmations to Transform Your Health Anxiety into Strength and Serenity

Spiritual Primate

Free Tools & Resources for Self-Development
https://spiritualprimate.com/

INTRODUCTION

In a world that often feels overwhelming and uncertain, our mental and physical health can take a toll. One common struggle many individuals face is health anxiety—an all-consuming fear of illness that can cripple even the strongest among us. But what if we could transform this anxiety into strength and serenity? What if we could harness the power of our minds to create a sense of empowerment and resilience? That's where affirmations come in.

Welcome to a journey of self-discovery and empowerment, where we will explore 50 empowering affirmations to transform your health anxiety into strength and serenity. These affirmations are not mere words; they are powerful tools that can reshape your mindset and help you navigate the challenges of health anxiety with grace and courage.

In the following pages, you will find a collection

of affirmations carefully crafted to address the specific fears and worries that often accompany health anxiety. From calming your racing thoughts to embracing self-compassion, each affirmation is designed to empower you to take control of your mental and physical well-being. So, let's embark on this transformative journey together and unlock the incredible potential within you.

UNDERSTANDING HEALTH ANXIETY: A COMPREHENSIVE EXPLORATION

What is Health Anxiety?

Health anxiety, also known as illness anxiety disorder or hypochondria, is a psychological condition characterized by excessive worry and fear about having a serious medical condition. If you constantly find yourself preoccupied with thoughts about your health, obsessively checking for signs and symptoms, seeking reassurance from doctors or loved ones, and experiencing significant distress even when medical tests come back negative, you may be dealing with health anxiety.

The Cognitive and Behavioral Aspects of Health Anxiety

Health anxiety is rooted in cognitive and behavioral patterns that contribute to the development and maintenance of this condition. The cognitive aspect involves distorted thinking patterns, such as catastrophizing (assuming the worst outcome), selectively focusing on bodily sensations, and misinterpreting benign symptoms as indicators of a severe illness. The behavioral aspect includes frequent doctor visits, seeking unnecessary medical tests, and engaging in excessive health-related research.

Causes and Risk Factors

While the exact causes of health anxiety are not fully understood, several factors can contribute to its development. These may include:

Previous traumatic experiences: If you have experienced a severe illness or witnessed a loved one's struggle with a medical condition, it may increase your likelihood of developing health anxiety.

Personality traits: Certain personality traits, such as being highly neurotic or having a tendency towards perfectionism, may make you more susceptible to health anxiety.

Family history: There is evidence to suggest that health anxiety can run in families, indicating a potential genetic component.

Impact on Daily Life

Health anxiety can significantly impact your daily life, affecting your overall well-being, relationships, and ability to function effectively. The constant worry and fear may lead to social isolation, difficulty concentrating on tasks, and interference with work or academic performance. It can also strain relationships as loved ones may struggle to understand and support your concerns.

Differentiating Health Anxiety from Genuine Medical Conditions

It is important to differentiate health anxiety from actual medical conditions. While health anxiety involves excessive worry about having a serious illness, genuine medical conditions are based on objective medical evidence and professional diagnosis. It is essential to consult a healthcare professional to accurately assess and address any health concerns.

Treatment and Management Strategies

Effective treatment for health anxiety typically involves a combination of therapeutic interventions. Cognitive-behavioral therapy (CBT) is commonly used, helping you identify and challenge negative thinking patterns, develop coping skills, and gradually reduce safety behaviors. Medication, such as selective serotonin reuptake inhibitors (SSRIs), may also be prescribed in some cases.

In addition to professional help, you can also adopt self-help strategies to manage health anxiety. These may include:

Limiting health-related internet searches: Constantly searching for symptoms online can increase anxiety and reinforce irrational beliefs.

Engaging in relaxation techniques: Practices like deep breathing exercises, mindfulness, and yoga can help reduce anxiety levels.

Seeking social support: Sharing your concerns with trusted loved ones can provide reassurance and a sense of perspective.

Engaging in pleasurable activities: Focusing on activities you enjoy can distract your mind from health-related worries and promote overall well-being.

Overcoming Health Anxiety

Overcoming health anxiety is a gradual process that requires commitment and persistence. By seeking professional help, implementing effective strategies, and challenging irrational thoughts, you can learn to manage your anxiety and regain control over your life. Remember, you are not alone, and with the right support, you can overcome health anxiety and live a fulfilling and healthy life.

In conclusion, health anxiety is a psychological condition characterized by excessive worry and fear about having a serious medical condition. It can significantly impact your daily life, relationships, and overall well-being. However, with appropriate treatment, self-help strategies, and support, you can overcome health anxiety and regain control over your thoughts and emotions. Remember to seek professional help and surround yourself with a supportive network of loved ones.

HARNESSING THE POWER OF POSITIVE AFFIRMATIONS: RELIEVING HEALTH ANXIETY

Understanding Positive Affirmations

Positive affirmations are powerful statements that are intentionally designed to shape and influence your thoughts, beliefs, and behaviors. They are concise, positive statements that reflect the reality you desire to create. By repeating these affirmations regularly, you can reprogram your subconscious mind and transform your perception of yourself and the world around you.

The Benefits of Positive Affirmations for Health Anxiety

Health anxiety, also known as illness anxiety disorder or hypochondria, is a condition characterized by excessive worry and fear about having a serious medical condition. This debilitating anxiety can lead to a constant state of distress, affecting your overall well-being and quality of life. Incorporating positive affirmations into your daily routine can have significant benefits in relieving health anxiety.

Shifting Focus: Positive affirmations help shift your focus from negative and anxious thoughts to positive and empowering ones. By consciously choosing to focus on affirmations that promote health, well-being, and resilience, you can redirect your attention away from anxiety-inducing thoughts.

Replacing Negative Beliefs: Health anxiety often stems from deep-seated negative beliefs about health and illness. Positive affirmations offer an opportunity to challenge and replace these negative beliefs with positive, empowering ones. By repeating affirmations that reinforce your innate strength and ability to overcome challenges, you can gradually rewire your mind to embrace a healthier perspective.

Cultivating Self-Compassion: Health anxiety can often be accompanied by self-criticism and self-blame. Positive affirmations provide a platform for cultivating self-compassion and self-acceptance. By nurturing a kind and supportive inner dialogue, you can develop a sense of inner peace, which can help alleviate anxiety.

Incorporating Positive Affirmations into Your Daily Life

Identify Your Triggers: Reflect on the specific triggers that exacerbate your health anxiety. These triggers may include certain medical symptoms, news articles, or experiences. Once you identify your triggers, create affirmations that counteract these negative thoughts and fears. For example, if you fear a specific symptom, create an affirmation such as "I am healthy and resilient, and my body knows how to heal itself."

Create Personalized Affirmations: Tailor your affirmations to your specific needs and desires. Use words that resonate with you and reflect the positive reality you wish to create. For example, if you struggle with anxiety about your physical health, affirmations such as "I am in control of my health and well-being" or "I trust my body's ability to heal and thrive" can be powerful in shifting your mindset.

Consistency is Key: Repeat your affirmations consistently throughout the day. You can write them down, say them out loud, or even create recordings to listen to during moments of anxiety. Consistency helps reinforce the new beliefs you are cultivating and strengthens the neural pathways associated with positive thinking.

Visualize Your Affirmations: In addition to repeating affirmations, visualize yourself already embodying the reality you desire. Imagine yourself feeling calm, healthy, and in control. Visualization enhances the impact of affirmations by creating a vivid mental image of your desired outcome.

Affirmations on the Go: Incorporate affirmations into your daily routine. Write them on sticky notes and place them where you'll see them often, such as on your bathroom mirror, computer screen, or phone wallpaper. By integrating affirmations into your environment, you provide constant reminders to focus on positive thoughts.

The Power of Your Mindset

Your mindset plays a crucial role in your overall well-being. By cultivating a positive mindset through the practice of positive affirmations, you can significantly reduce health anxiety and improve your mental and physical health. Remember that change takes time and consistency, so be patient with yourself as you embark on this journey. Embrace the power of positive affirmations, and watch as your thoughts, beliefs, and ultimately, your life transform for the better.

Ultimately, it is up to you to take control of your thoughts and beliefs. By embracing positive affirmations, you have the power to relieve health anxiety, cultivate a positive mindset, and create a life filled with joy, resilience, and well-being. Start today, and witness the transformative power of affirmations unfold in your life.

POSITIVE AFFIRMATIONS FOR HEALTH ANXIETY

1. I am stronger than my worries about my health.

This affirmation is meant to empower you. It's reminding you that your strength exceeds your health-related worries.

2. My body is healthy, and I am grateful.

This affirmation encourages gratitude for your health, which can help shift your focus from anxiety to positivity.

3. I trust the natural healing processes of my body.

This affirmation promotes trust in your body's

natural ability to heal itself, reducing unnecessary worry about your health.

4. I am in control of my thoughts, not my health anxieties.

This affirmation helps you remember that you are in control of your thoughts, even when dealing with health anxiety.

5. I release all negative energy and fears about my health.

This affirmation acts as a mantra for you to release your fears and negative thoughts about your health.

6. Every breath I take is a step towards a healthier me.

By focusing on the act of breathing, this affirmation helps you to stay present and grounded, reducing your health anxieties.

7. I choose to nourish my body with positive thoughts and actions.

This affirmation encourages you to actively choose positivity and healthy actions over worry and negativity.

8. I am filled with energy and vitality.

This affirmation serves to reinforce your belief in your own vitality and wellness, countering health anxiety.

9. I am patient with my body and my health.

This affirmation reminds you to show patience and understanding towards your body, reducing the stress that comes with health anxiety.

10. I am in tune with my body's needs and capabilities.

This affirmation encourages you to listen closely to your body and understand its needs, reducing the tendency to panic over perceived health issues.

11. I am learning to accept my body as it is.

This affirmation promotes body acceptance, which can ease your health anxiety by helping you accept your body's natural state.

12. I am resilient and can handle my health concerns.

This affirmation encourages you to believe in your resilience when dealing with health concerns.

13. I trust my doctors and their expertise.

This affirmation helps you to put trust in your healthcare providers, reducing the anxiety that can come from doubting their advice.

14. I am moving towards a healthier future.

This affirmation reminds you that every step you take is towards a healthier future, reducing the anxiety of uncertainty.

15. My health does not define me.

This affirmation helps you remember that your worth is not defined by your health status, which can help reduce health anxiety.

16. I am capable of managing my health anxiety.

This affirmation empowers you to take control of your health anxiety.

17. I am free from my health worries.

This affirmation helps you visualize a state of being free from health worries, which can be therapeutic.

18. I am choosing to focus on positivity and health.

This affirmation encourages you to actively choose positivity and health over worry and anxiety.

19. I respect my body and treat it well.

This affirmation reminds you of the importance of treating your body with respect, which can reduce health anxiety.

20. I release the need to worry about my health.

This affirmation serves as a mantra to help you let go of your need to worry about your health.

21. I am in charge of how I feel and today I choose health and happiness.

This affirmation reminds you that you can choose how you feel, encouraging you to choose health and happiness over anxiety.

22. I am confident in my body's abilities and strength.

This affirmation boosts your confidence in your body's abilities, helping to reduce health anxiety.

23. I am at peace with my body and health.

This affirmation promotes a sense of peace and acceptance with your body and health status, alleviating health anxiety.

24. My health is improving every day.

This affirmation encourages a positive outlook towards your health progress, reducing health anxiety.

25. I am not my illness. I am a person independent of my health concerns.

This affirmation helps to separate your identity from your health concerns, easing health anxiety.

26. I am more than capable of taking care of my health.

This affirmation instills confidence in your ability to manage your health effectively.

27. I am doing my best and that is enough.

This affirmation reassures you that your best effort is enough, reducing the pressure and anxiety surrounding your health.

28. I am deserving of good health and happiness.

This affirmation emphasizes your deservingness of good health and happiness, promoting a positive self-image.

29. I am capable of making positive health decisions.

This affirmation boosts your confidence in your ability to make healthy decisions, reducing health anxiety.

30. I am surrounded by love and support on my health journey.

This affirmation encourages a sense of community and support, which can reduce feelings of isolation related to health anxiety.

31. I am proactive about my health.

This affirmation promotes proactive behavior in maintaining and improving your health instead of dwelling on health worries.

32. I am focusing on the now, not worrying about the future.

This affirmation helps you to stay present and reduce anxiety about potential future health issues.

33. I am letting go of fear and choosing to live in courage.

This affirmation encourages you to let go of fear, replacing it with courage, which can help in managing health anxiety.

34. I am a warrior and can handle anything that comes my way.

This affirmation boosts your confidence and resilience, reminding you of your strength in facing health concerns.

35. I am in harmony with my body.

This affirmation promotes a sense of harmony and peace with your body, reducing health anxiety.

36. I am trusting my body to do its job.

This affirmation encourages trust in your body's natural functions and healing processes, reducing health anxiety.

37. I am prioritizing self-care and mental wellness.

This affirmation emphasizes the importance of self-care and mental wellness in maintaining physical health and reducing anxiety.

38. I am accepting of my body's limitations and capabilities.

This affirmation promotes acceptance of your body's limitations, which can help reduce health anxiety by setting realistic expectations.

39. I am focusing on the positives in my life.

This affirmation encourages a positive mindset, which can help reduce health anxiety.

40. I am taking steps to improve my health every day.

This affirmation reminds you that you're actively working on improving your health, reducing the anxiety of feeling stuck or helpless.

41. I am not alone in my health journey.

This affirmation reassures you that you are not alone in your health journey, which can help reduce feelings of isolation related to health anxiety.

42. I am choosing to live a healthy and balanced life.

This affirmation promotes the choice of living a balanced life, which can reduce health anxiety by promoting overall wellbeing.

43. I am grateful for the good health I enjoy.

This affirmation encourages gratitude for the health you do have, shifting your focus from anxiety to positivity.

44. I am dedicated to living a healthy lifestyle.

This affirmation emphasizes your commitment to health, reducing anxiety by reminding you of your dedication.

45. I am capable of overcoming health challenges.

This affirmation boosts your confidence in your ability to tackle health challenges, reducing health anxiety.

46. I am responsible for my health and wellness.

This affirmation promotes taking responsibility for your health and wellness, reducing anxiety by encouraging a sense of control.

47. I am focusing on healing and recovery.

This affirmation directs your focus towards healing and recovery, reducing anxiety by promoting a proactive approach to health.

48. I am finding joy in my health journey.

This affirmation encourages finding joy in your health journey, promoting positivity and reducing health anxiety.

49. I am deserving of a life free from health

anxiety.

This affirmation reinforces your deservingness of a life free from health anxiety, promoting a positive self-image.

50. I am embracing my health with love and kindness.

This affirmation encourages you to approach your health with love and kindness, reducing anxiety by promoting a compassionate approach.

FINAL WORDS

As we come to the end of this empowering journey, we invite you to reflect on the immense power that lies within your mind. You have discovered how affirmations can shift your perspective, calm your anxiety, and foster strength and serenity in the face of health-related worries. By embracing these affirmations, you have taken a proactive step towards reclaiming control over your mental and physical well-being.

But remember, transformation is an ongoing process. It requires commitment, practice, and self-compassion. As you continue on your journey, let the lessons learned here serve as a guiding light in moments of doubt or fear. Remember that you have the strength within you to overcome any obstacle that comes your way.

So, as you move forward, ask yourself: How will you use the power of affirmations to shape your future? How will you harness the strength and serenity you have cultivated to not only conquer health anxiety but also embrace a life of vitality and joy?

Take these empowering affirmations with you, carry them in your heart, and let them fuel your transformation. You possess the potential to create a life filled with strength, serenity, and a deep appreciation for the incredible resilience of the human spirit. Embrace it, nurture it, and watch as your journey unfolds with newfound purpose and grace.

MORE SELF-DEVELOPMENT TOOLS

Congratulations on finishing this book!

We hope you enjoyed the journey and learned something valuable along the way. But remember, personal growth is a lifelong journey, and there's always more to discover.

That's why we recommend checking out **spiritualprimate.com** for a wealth of tools and resources for your ongoing self-development.

At Spiritual Primate, you'll find all the tools you need for personal growth and transformation to help you unlock your full potential.

Whether you're looking to deepen your spiritual

practice, improve your relationships, or enhance your career, spiritualprimate.com has something for everyone.

We believe that everyone has the power to create the life they want, and we're here to help you achieve your goals.

We look forward to supporting you on your path to self-discovery and growth.

www.ingramcontent.com/pod-product-compliance
Lightning Source LLC
Chambersburg PA
CBHW060908260726
48661CB00008B/3539